The Si___ _____ __ Happiness

An Essential Mindful Guide on How to be Happy and Transform Your Life into a Blissful Journey

Anuradha Garg

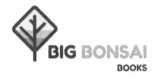

BIG BONSAI
BOOKS

Published by BIG BONSAI BOOKS

The Six Pillars of Happiness

Copyright © 2017 by Big Bonsai Books

ISBN -13: 978-1544673851

ISBN -10: 154467385X

Cover Designed by Rachel Pepperberg, German Creative.

Printed in the United States of America.

Dedicated to you

May The Six Pillars bring you love and

happiness for your entire existence.

There is no duty we so much underrate as the duty of being happy.

- Robert Louis Stevenson

CONTENT

Introduction

What if you have to look back at your life some day and find nothing that could cheer you up? It so happened to me as I started receiving the "distress call". As I wandered in search of happiness and peace, I observe that happiness remains as elusive as proof of life on Mars in our lives.

Treading on broken pieces

It was fourth consecutive night that I have cried to sleep. As I saw myself in the mirror next morning, a glowing pretty face looked back. I could not believe that somebody so broken inside can look so normal.

I walked into the office to be greeted by my bubbly colleague.

"Hey, how are you?"Mary chirped.

"I am good" I replied in a well-practiced tone.

We were to discuss the new project that we were about to start. But then all of a sudden my hands started to shake uncontrollably. Thankfully, Mary was still rummaging through the papers. She did not notice anything.

But, how can it be? It has been just a week since I have received my "distress call". I have not been able to feel my usual self since then.

It was about to clock midnight, my resolve to sleep early seem to fail again as I surfed through the television channels. Thereafter, I felt a deep anguish inside my heart out of the blue. Or maybe not all of a sudden, it has been building for some time now.

Michael's parting words rung in my ears, "You could have come to my brother's wedding; you could have met my entire family."And then my own sobbing shaky reply succeeded the angry voice, "I would not have known anybody there."

I felt hurt when I remembered that my best friend Pamela took her other friend to a music concert. It even hurt more when I recollected that she did not even share this with me and I got to know it from someone else. I shook my head and tried to concentrate on the television.

As speed skaters rolled on the ice to glory at the world championship organized at Nanjing, China, my own adventure cut short due to lack of funds came weighing down on my chest. As I gasped for breath, tears came rolling down my cheeks. I closed my eyes and took a deep breath. But, there was no respite from the swirling memories that were rushing into my mind.

I also caught a glimpse of my appraisal that has happened a week ago. The crushing declaration that I have not been promoted in the third year as well sickened me further. Since then, I have not been the same. I have been getting "distress calls" every now and then.

Between distress and disappointment, I started finding my broken pieces so that I can weave them back together for a happy life. I knew if I would continue my life like this I might end up popping pills for depression. So I began my hunt for self-actualization and inner peace. I started my hunt and received wisdom from various psychologists, experts, wellness gurus, and counselors. Each one of them had a vision of their own and had something to contribute as remedies to my so-called 'disease'.

My experience taught me that these six pillars can bring about a sea change in the level of contentment in your life. You can be a young girl or a housewife, a businessman or a retired banker, but you always have problems in life, the key is to know how to deal with them. We all know the "grandma's guidance" is that happiness lies in giving not asking, happiness lies in feeding the poor, happiness lies in saving the animals, happiness lies in respecting your elders and so on. I strongly agree with them but this is not the solution to our modern lives' mess. We need to have some easy and quick solutions which 'really' work and they work all throughout our lives. They should be like a magic spell that always work for us every time.

I can assure you that I have my magic spell and I have found results. Today not only I am a contented and confident girl but also I have done very well in my career. I am working at flourishing of a boutique consulting firm. I have started giving group counseling to young college students and working class people. I have learned various skills like acting at presentations, handling crisis and speaking French. I am basically a newer and a better person for sure.

The laid-out tactics are bound to help achieve both personal and professional goals by improving relationships, developing a positive attitude and becoming connected with inner self.

It all begins now.

Pillar One: Break the 'E' bubble

If I have to point the biggest reason for my unhappiness, it would be a disappointment. Perhaps, if I have to state one reason for everybody's distress in this world, it would still be the same.

None of us are free from disappointments that arise from us not meeting the set targets. Whether it is missing a promotion or being ignored by a best friend or being hurt by a beloved, the end result is always a disappointment. But, to eradicate disappointment, we need to know the source of its origin.

Every disappointment is well rooted in our expectations. We have certain expectations in our lives, if that does not work out in our thought-out manner, we are filled with disappointment.

Relationships and 'E'xpectations

We all expect a certain amount of love and care in all relationships that we form whether at home or as we grow, from our friends or romantic relationships and also from our workplace as well in the form of respect and support if not love as such. Although these relationships are supposed to contribute to our happy life, it does not happen many times. Each relationship suffers from setbacks of conflicts, disagreements, and misunderstandings. As a result, relationships turn out to be our source of distress and mental trauma as contrary to their stated objective.

The strife with Pamela made me shed more tears than I would not have imagined on missing any of the concerts on this earth. But, it was not because of the gap in the relationship that I felt hurt and isolated. It was because of my expectations arising out of the friendship that I was depressed.

Whenever we become close to anyone, we expect them to behave in a certain manner so that we feel cared. However, a person does not always meet our expectations for him or her. This results in an uncontrollable agitation and irritation with that person even if his mistake was a puny one.

Thus, it is very important to let go of expectations so that we can enjoy the perks of a relationship without needing to hold it tight.

Then, the question arises as to how can we let go of expectations, is it not as natural as feeling happy or sad?

Only if we constantly practice the art of **"putting ourselves into the shoes of another person"**, we eventually develop empathy. This deeper understanding of people will help us to let go of grudges that arise every time a person behaves in a manner we do not like.

In this manner, we not only develop understanding into our relationships, but also we become better at creating boundaries in our relationships. This helps us in making relationships to last longer. It will also lead to attracting right kind of people into our lives rather than having acquaintances who only wish to use us for their ulterior motives.

I was expecting to be invited to a bachelor party of a friend. However, when he forgot to invite me, I felt devastated. I could no longer maintain the so-called friendship with him. I never tried to find out the reason for his behavior as he could have been very busy with his wedding preparations. As I let go of expectations, I would turn up at important events of my close friends even without bothering about invitations. Or at least try to understand the reason behind their behavior before I severe ties with them.

Being free from expectations also leads to being non-judgmental as we do not expect a person to behave in a certain manner and thus, we do not label a behavior as wrong or right. Such non-judgmental mindset is extremely beneficial in interacting with the world. We tend to gain so much when we do not limit ourselves by certain set standards.

I have been able to interact with people of all kinds and people of all ideologies when I stopped having a fixed mindset. My relationships with my colleagues, my friends, and even strangers got better when I started listening to them to understand rather than to judge or feel envious. I could not see why Pamela would ever again take any other friend to any concert!

Sometimes, it even sounds paradoxical to not having any expectations in a relationship because after all we are supposed to gain something from our connections with different people of our lives. But, when we form connections just to achieve love and affection, there would not be an expectation of receiving anything back. In such a scenario, whatever love and affection we receive back is more than enough for us because we are not expecting anything back.

It is like receiving interest money from an account we did not know provides any interest. Everything will be a bonus to our happiness account!

Goals and 'E'xpectations

I expected myself to rise to middle management in three years of my job. And when it did not happen, I was devastated. Suddenly, I could only see people who got promoted to the level I have set my eyes on. My despair grew deeper.

As in relationships, we do set our expectations on different goals we formulate in our lives. And we are full of negative anxiety and anguish when those goals do not materialize. So, does that mean we should not have any aim in our lives? Of course not. How else will we progress in life? The idea is to give our hundred percent efforts to the goal. If it materializes, then all is well. If it does not materialize, we can move to set another goal in life rather than brood over what we could have achieved.

My aim to achieve the goal of being an entrepreneur is hampered by my anxiety to be a successful entrepreneur. If I stop worrying about the end result, I can focus all my energies on giving my best to the task of setting up the enterprise, connecting with prospective customers, finding diligent employees and providing a good product. The venture might turn out to be a success or failure. But, I would have at least worked to make it best rather than constantly worrying about its success.

So, as long as we are giving our personal best to whatever task we undertake, we should not be worried about results.

Even when we do not get what we want, we have learned one more way that it does not work. Ha Ha, Cliched!! But that's actually true. When we develop the learning mindset rather than focusing on gains, we will only progress in our lives. All the work we will do to achieve the goal will not be wasted because it will lead to a better form of us. So, even if we do not gain the desired promotion or any another goal, we will still be happy as we would be moving closer to the bigger goals of our life. The work on establishing a startup would make me grow whether I have succeeded or failed. It will also help me in my future endeavors.

We spend a lot of time working towards a goal rather than the achievement of the goal. In many ways, the journey becomes more important than the destination. Thus, it is important to detach ourselves from outcomes so that we can enjoy the process of learning rather than constantly running after targets. In this manner, we will gain happiness in the intervening time as well which we could have wasted on nervously anticipating about our outcomes.

I could now work with a growth mindset rather than solely focused on outcomes, which has not only improved my inner satisfaction but also the quality of my efforts resulting in outperforming in my goals.

Therefore, we need to break free from the chains of expectations to progress in our life, whether by means of better relationships or fulfilled goals. We will let go of the end result. We will be happy whether we succeed or not in our set goal. Also, our relationships will become gratifying as we will become more understanding and non-judgmental.

Break Free from the chains of expectation to progress in our life.

Pillar Two: Show me the light

Most of us are privileged enough to live a life away from adversaries that many people experience on this planet. We have never inhabited a war stricken area, we have never gone to sleep on an empty stomach or we have not met with any serious accident. But, still, most of us appear to be the most unfortunate, unthankful beings on the face of the earth.

It is our tendency to adopt negativity rather than framing positive responses that ruin the joy of living. We tend to look at glass half-empty rather than glass half-full. We keep on comparing ourselves with lives of other people, sapping ourselves of strength that could have been used to achieve positive results. This will help us in making decisions that will strengthen our life rather than being driven by fate.

According to a study conducted in 2000 by four researchers Fredrickson, Mancuso, Branigan, & Tugade, positive emotions were found capable of undoing the cardiovascular after-effects of negative events. Researchers first showed the participants a clip inducing fear, a thereafter different set of participants were shown four different clips with two of them inducing positivity and other two inducing sadness/neutrality. It was found that the groups shown the positive clips shower the fastest recovery as compared with those shown negative clips.

Therefore, it is important to **"cultivate positivity"** so that we can enjoy every day of our life. We need to keep our good head on our shoulders to storm any turmoil of our lives.

Tracing inspirations

Now, the question arises as to how we can make ourselves positive about our life amidst its ups and downs. We need to look for inspirations that exist around us. The world is full of exemplary examples of people who have survived odds and what more even emerged stronger through those odds. If we look at them, follow them and try to emulate them, we will have the inspiration to beat the difficulties of our lives.

People who have survived difficulties like Nelson Mandela are great examples to emulate in tough times. How he spent 27 years in an abysmal state and still had the courage to fight for a cause can show us light even in the darkest of times. We might never experience the extent of his agony but if a fellow human being can remain positive in such a situation, then we definitely can be positive.

Many sportspersons who set themselves apart every single day like Michael Phelps, who despite suffering from attention disorder at an early age, continues to make a mark at Olympics. His winning of 28 medals has rewritten the history of the mother of all sporting events. The ability of such sportsperson to get up every time they fall on the field is a testimony to the spirit of human being. However, some exceptional athletes go a step forward. They use their failures as stepping stone to give a better performance in their races. Similarly, we can use our failures as a propellant to succeed more vigorously rather than getting defeated by them.

Michael Jordan used his failures effectively to emerge as a formidable competitor. He has dropped off the team during his initial days of playing basketball. The list that did not have his name continued to drive him unless he achieved success on the same court. He counts his failures to be his blessings that led to his extraordinary success.

Following inspirations can help us in feeling positive in down times as we will be able to see that there are people around the world who are defeating odds every single day through the strength of their spirit. Inspirations continue to be our guiding light whenever darkness threatens to engulf us.

As I started following the journey of such people, I found that my troubles are laughable. I have been able to take myself less seriously and enjoy myself without constantly feeling sorry for myself as there are people in this world who are doing tougher tasks than me.

Building strength

It is natural to be bogged down by negativity especially if we go through adverse times, have to deal with difficult people or encounter tough situations. However, human beings have been given a gift to choose their response to a situation rather than letting the situation overwhelm them. We need to set up small goals so that achieving them can give us a sense of confidence and strength over time. For example: If we have set up a target to get up at 6 AM every day to run 2 miles, we will not feel like doing it for a couple of days. But, if we constantly push ourselves to do it for a couple of days, we will develop a resolve to meet our targets by looking at our achievement in hindsight.

According to research, it takes 17 days to break a bad habit. It can only happen if a person sets realistic goals and he or she is able to break self-limiting beliefs. Then, the person will be able to get rid of negative behavior patterns.

We can also build our internal reserve of strength by following a disciplined lifestyle. We need to constantly follow a regime of exercise and have regular sleeping patterns. In that manner, we will gather stamina to endure hardships that may arise in our day-to-day lives without letting them overpower us. This stamina will help in the achievement of greater heights as bigger goals will require harder efforts.

We also inculcate strength in our minds if we follow a set of values consistently. We need to be fair to others and to ourselves to truly bring justice in our everyday interactions with other people. This will lead to a strength of character which we will enable a greater control over our actions. We will make more thorough decisions rather than following impulses.

Oliver Twist characterizes someone with a strong value system. He was constantly mistreated in the story. He was forced to work under dismal conditions in the workhouse. Thereafter, he was sold off to an undertaker just for asking for some extra food. As he runs away to escape from wretched conditions, he had to cope up with thieves. However, he did not lose his strength to believe in people. Towards the end of the story, he gave his wicked half-brother his property so that he can prosper in life. He even went to soothe Fagin, one of the culprits who caused Oliver suffering, at the time of his hanging.

Both internal and external strength is necessary to lead a happy life. Following a disciplined routine not only in terms of activities but also in our interactions with people will lead to enhanced strength in life. Such an emancipated way of living is bound to create a peaceful life. The tasks that looked daunting to me earlier has become as easy as have developed ways to harness my inner strength. It has also improved my levels of fitness as I could now utilize my time in going to the gym rather than watching television.

Practicing compassion

It is the mandate of the universe that we feel uplifted when we help our fellow human beings in times of distress. If we practice compassion in our daily lives, we can become stronger internally. But, it is not as easily achieved as it is stated. We need to develop acceptance of people before we can fully understand the true meaning of compassion. And that can come only through continuously helping people.

A leader who demonstrated acceptance of people of all kinds can be seen in Martin Luther King. He fought for an equal society without resorting to violence. He inspired and influenced million of people to create a compassionate society. His work for equality of people also earned him Nobel Peace Prize. His dedication to the cause was evident from the fact that he even used his prize money to continue his fight for justice.

We need to see the purpose of aiding people in meeting their goals rather than competing with them. It is not difficult to find purpose in a world full of suffering. Maybe what we can do is not big enough to hit the headlines, but if it is making a positive difference in anybody's life, it will bring purpose into our lives. It could be as simple as sharing the load of a person struggling through loss of a loved one. Such a mindset will create a joyful existence for us as well as for others.

Mother Teresa enlightened the world through her work for humanity. She served poor and downtrodden people to bring joy to the most inaccessible corners of the world. Her compassion for wretched and sick people still remind the world the power of miracles.

Compassion can make us a better human being as we will be more aware of sufferings of others even if we do not go through any adversaries. It will lead to improvement in our relationships as we will be more tolerant of our friends or our colleagues or spouses. It will also lead to the creation of a better world as the world will be filled with hope and peace.

My humane treatment of my fellow beings has won me many friendships, association with wonderful people and a greater sense of existence. The feeling that I can make difference in the life of others has amplified my belief in life.

Therefore, positivity has the power to brighten our lives, lives of our loved ones and lives of our fellow beings. We just need to continuously look for inspirational role models, have a disciplined life to create strength and have a compassionate outlook to help and uplift others.

Find inspiration for your goal, build your strength and be compassionate towards people.

Pillar Three: Silence Please– Power of solitude

Happiness is dependent upon the company of wonderful people in our lives. We have read it, heard it and ingrained it in us as gospel truth.

I had to constantly talk and search for friends or potential friends. I had to keep company to keep myself happy. But, as I lay awake on one of the night's cryings, I could not think of calling even one of my acquaintances. As I searched more desperately for the company, I felt more and more lonely. What if speech makes us feel lonely rather than befriended? What if keeping more company make us lose ourselves? We often lose touch with ourselves when we adopt noise rather than silence, as being comfortable with silence requires depth and strength.

Maybe it is only in silence that we can understand our own selves. It is only in silence that we can be comfortable with ourselves. There cannot be a better friend than oneself. And silence can help us find peace with our own selves.

As per experiment conducted by biologist Imke Kirste, silence proved to be conducive to growth in the brain. She undertook a study to measure the effect of various sounds on brains of mice. She subjected mice to four types of sounds: music, baby mouse call, white noise, and silence. She discovered that silence led to the development of a cell in the hippocampus area of the brain. Therefore, silence proved to be even more advantageous than listening to music.

Silence can also help us in avoiding various problems in our social life. The ability to keep our mouth shut is extremely beneficial in not indulging in gossips, backbiting and malicious talks. These habits hurt personal relationship when we gossip incessantly.

Silence is as essential as speech in keeping our relationships enriching. We breach the trust of people when we are not able to keep matters confidential. If we are not able to keep the conversations with other people private, people will not feel comfortable in opening their heart to us. In addition, silence enriches our listening skills as we do not feel a continuous urge to speak to connect with anybody.

Abraham Lincoln remains one of the most prominent figures in American history. He has been credited with the eradication of slavery during his presidency. He was known to be a great orator who could deliver speeches that mobilized the audience. But, he was also quiet by nature. His ability to remain silent not only provided him the ability to understand him but also to connect with masses.

Reading and Solitude

We can only feel the silence in its purest form when we are cut out from the real world. Reading provides a great escape from the world by imbibing us into the world of stories. Reading is counted as one of the best habits as it provides us an opportunity to connect with ourselves. We are no longer part of the social setup where we need to play our role to meet social obligations. We can let our imagination loose to understand and experience different perspectives by remaining still in silence. Such a silence is not disturbing like loneliness; rather it empowers us by providing knowledge and wisdom.

When we make friends with books, we do not need constant companions to ward off loneliness. We feel happy and contented with ourselves. In such a situation, we seek company only to add more colors to our lives rather than to avoid loneliness. Therefore, reading helps us in seeking more fulfilling relationships as we embrace our own selves.

Needless to say, reading also helps us in grooming us as an individual. We start having a viewpoint on things we have never experienced. We can easily converse with different people on different topics. We become more enjoyable as a company. Although we may seek silence then, but we become better friends as we are at peace with ourselves.

Writing and Solitude

We do not need to be a writer to pen down our confusions, our sadness, and our struggles. Writing down our problems is the easiest way to be face to face with our innermost thoughts. This exercise can help us in sorting out most of the struggles of our life as most of the times even we are not aware of issues that are bothering us.

Thus, it is important to regularly write down our thoughts and feelings so that we can live a life full of self-awareness rather than being driven by circumstances. Writing ensures we are enjoying time spent in our own company as we are all alone while penning downs our thoughts. It also helps us keeping a track of how we have evolved over years as we keep a journal of our activities.

Travelling and Solitude

Going to new places can be deeply enriching as it helps us in discovering new facets of our personality. We discover so much about ourselves when we travel to unknown spheres. We meet different kinds of people and terrains as we travel which helps us in learning the art of adapting. Travelling also helps us to be open-minded as we are just supposed to enjoy the moment rather than analyzing events as we usually do with our daily life.

Especially if we travel on our own, we will be founding a great friend in ourselves. It gives us an opportunity to understand ourselves in different setups when we travel across areas, cultures, and people.

Yoga and Solitude

Meditation and yoga are other powerful tools to be in sync with the inner self. When we do yoga, we need to gain control over our senses and breathing to attain a feeling of relaxation. These exercises help us gain harmony with our inner vibes so that we become more aware of our problems and anxieties.

Such a heightened sense of ourselves is bound to help in improving our well-being as we can work on solving our issues.

Therefore, we should continuously pursue activities that enable us to become our own best friend by spending quality time with ourselves. When we pursue such activities, we no longer seek comfort from others as we become our own biggest source of comfort and peace.

Become your own best friend by indulging in activities that provide solitude.

Pillar Four: The Better Gender

It is ironical that girls have been given the right to create life but they are fighting for their rights all their life. So, we tend to find the grumpiest human beings among women. And we wonder why they are grumpy. Maybe it is that time of the month.

But, we do not wonder that maybe they are not succeeding in their fight for equal rights. There is still cry over equal representation of women in corporate leadership, politics, and households but women are sulking as they know it is not true even after centuries of fighting. However, if they have a lot of being unhappy about, they also have the ability to celebrate themselves.

Females are stronger because they are more aware of themselves. They have better ability to regulate their emotions as they are more in touch with their bodies. They have the power to read and understand others much better than their male counterparts. But, that can only happen if they develop the power of womanhood.

Adrienne Rich portrays the power of a true feminist. Her writings bring forth the problem of male dominance in American society. Her poems illustrated how women are traditionally subjugated. She narrated the bondage of married women, unnecessary burdens of daughter-in-law and persuasion of women to recognize their own power.

So, how does one develops the power of womanhood? That can happen if we constantly practice real feminism. Real feminism demands that women work hard to achieve their goals even if it means that women need to endure more than their male counterparts. If men can do something, women need to prove that they can do so wearing heels.

There are also a great number of men who display real feminism by understanding concerns of females even better than many females of this world.

Nullifying dominance and abuse

The male dominance is as prevalent in this era as it was hundred years ago. Every day, we hear news about domestic violence, violence against women over trivial issues and abject treatment of women. It stems from the mindset that still considers women as a property rather than an equal human being.

It affects the happiness of both the genders as neither men nor women feel accomplished in such a scenario. Men need to recognize that empowering women only leads to a better life for both as women have intrinsic qualities at managing certain tasks. Similarly, women need to recognize their true potential rather than acting as inferior to men.

Sexual offense or molestation is more common in the world than we will care to admit. It is essential that men respect the consent of women rather than treating them as objects of pleasure. Women need to identify that they are more than their bodies. They must exalt the ideology of upholding their honor when they are not stopped by baseless allegations on the character.

Erin Andrews is a classic example of the suffering of a woman even when she was a victim of peeping in a hotel. Her stalker posted her video online just to earn some easy money. Hotel owners even suggested that her harassment had proved beneficial to her as she has progressed in her career due to the case. She continued to be taunted every day despite having done nothing wrong. It is important for both men and women to not point fingers of shame at women.

Happiness is having a mutual respect between two genders rather than suppression of one gender by another. Although it is impossible to end every instance of dominance and exploitation by an individual, we need to accept equality between genders in every facet of our life to increase the sense of contentment. Barack and Michelle are a couple that exudes respect in its every gesture. From holding an umbrella for his wife to waiting at the airport to pick her up and mentioning her in all speeches, Barack portrays respect for his wife even during his role of President.

Discarding fakeness

Then, there is fake feminism. Girls who want to have an easy access to everything because well, they are girls. These females dilute the fight of real women and men, for we know that real men are only those who treat females as just another gender. We need to discard females who raise pink flags, females who think they have a right to cheat on men because somebody cheated on them, females who do constant drama to get preferential treatment because they are just using feminism as an excuse to excuse themselves of any hard work.

We also cannot underestimate the dilution of real feminism by people who think bashing up men or degrading men is equivalent to feminism. Quite the contrary, real feminism demands end of suppression of one gender by another gender be it male or female.

There was a movement to include "Amendment "by feminists as early as the 1900s which read, "Equality of rights under the law shall not be denied or abridged by the United States or by any state on account of sex."

Although it was not ratified, it represents the correct ideology of true feminism. It demanded the equal treatment of both the sexes rather than demeaning of men or special privileges for women.

Happiness demands that we empower women by working towards abolishing fakeness that has crept into feminism. Both men and women need to work to ensure that they are not doing only lip service to bringing about a change that is very basic in nature. This change will positively affect our surroundings, resulting in a more fulfilling life.

Therefore, we must strive to ensure equality among genders by raising our voice against every instance of domination and abuse we encounter in our daily lives. Also, we need to correct the inequalities that have crept between genders by proactively working towards imbibing it as a way of life. This measure will ensure our long-term happiness as we feel more empowered with empowered women all around us.

Pursue respect and security of women to bring gender balance

Pillar Five: It runs in the blood

I was born to be a part of the family. However, over years, I have lost touch with them. My plush apartment at Texas has become my dwelling. Sometimes, I even felt better that way as I need not put up with their attempts at conditioning me anymore.

But, I traded my firm roots for a hollow space. I could no longer call them and cry out my sorrow. What if they did not understand me, what if they do not comprehend the complications of my professional life?

There is an intrinsic comfort in being with family. Those are the people who make us at ease with ourselves. So, it does not matter if we are succeeding or failing, if we are holding the spotlight or are pushed away to the background, they are always standing by our side.

The family is also the set of people who bring out the best in us by guiding us, grooming us and sometimes even taunting us so that we can reach our maximum potential. But, they are not always defined by our birth. We meet many people in our journey of life who make us shine even at the cost of personal sufferings. These may come in form of teachers, coaches, mentors or even strangers. However, we could do really well in life if we could hold our inner circle together even if we may not be able to repay everyone's debt.

Family

There cannot be an overemphasis on the importance of the relationship with our parents as a foundation in our lives. Parents bring us into the world, mold our personality and thought process during childhood, support us during adult life and keep us grounded during middle life. They provide us the basics of how to successfully guide our lives through various ups and downs. So, even if they have not encountered similar situations in their lives, we are equipped to deal with whatever the destiny sends our way.

However, as we grow up, we sometimes start devaluing the importance of their teachings as we become more knowledgeable or we feel that we could have been imparted more direction. But, we must remember that whatever success we achieve in our lives, it is only because of their good parenting. They have done their best to teach us most valuable lessons of our lives which will never fade, no matter what generation we belong to or how old we get.

We must keep ourselves connected to our parents to keep replenishing that source of wisdom. We must also be grateful to them for raising us with love and care. After all, it is only their imparted values that attract our future friends, partner and other significant relationships towards us.

Family values are most visible in families where one parent or both parents serve the armed forces. Even when a parent is away to serve the nation in a foreign land, the love for his/her family keeps them motivated to fight. Similarly, the family always keep the far-away stationed parent(s) in their thoughts for every occasion. The short get-togethers are full of bonding and love as each member of the family knows that their time together is little and precious.

Then, there are our siblings that build another core part of our families. Our siblings can be a great source of comfort in our lives as we share a very deep bonding of sharing same family values, having similar tastes and preferences and belonging to the same set of parents and relatives.

So, it is necessary that we maintain at least a functional bond with them. This will enable us to remain close to what we are. Also, blood is thicker than water as siblings are those to whom we can always reach out for help and support.

As I stay more in touch with my family, I feel closer to the joy and innocence of childhood. My inherent nature remains still the same, but I could now connect to how comfortable I felt when I was not shouldering unnecessary troubles.

Friends as family

We choose our family when we choose our friends. We make friends with whom we share our core values. We befriend those with whom we can connect and share our deepest secrets.

But, it is essential that we choose those people as our friends who really care about us. Just us true friends can enlighten our lives; fake friends can drag us to into dark spheres of depression and distress. That's why we should be mindful of people intending to be our friends. We need to ensure that they demand nothing more than our happiness when they agree to be our friends.

The power of true friendships can help us overcome any unhappiness. They help us in seeing better things about ourselves even when we cannot. They help us in laughing at our faults. They help us in encountering any difficulty or trouble of our lives. These friendships are to be nurtured just as our family. It does not matter how busy we are or how hectic our schedules are. We need to be in touch with our friends constantly to be in touch with our inner self as we cannot astray from our heart's truest desires if we keep ourselves connected to those who know us the best.

The friendship of Sherlock Holmes and Dr.Watson is an example of how friends can understand each other even without uttering a word. Their joint search for clues, collective fighting off villains and their support for each other in every circumstance shows the power of friendship.

True friendships are also rare and long-lasting. We cannot find people who understand even our silence too often. And these people stick with us over a long period of time so that we no longer could distinguish between our made up relationships and blood relationships.

Second family

As we get married, we become part of another family. Most of us are concerned with choosing a right life partner, but to feel contented in life, we also need to be concerned about choosing right second family.

The family of our partner defines not only the values of the family we would be part of but also affects the behavior of our partner. In most likeliness, the value system of our partner is defined by his/her family. The traits and attributes of the partner will be inherited from his/her family. Thus, it becomes essential to know his/her family to completely understand our partner.

Also, their behavior towards us is influenced by their family. Thus, relationships with partner's life become extremely important in having a successful marriage and a tension-free life.

If we enjoy good relationships with parents of our partner, we will be happier. It will not only ensure that our relationship with our partner strengthens but also give us the benefit of having another set of parents.

Therefore, it is indispensable that we keep our house in order. This can only be done by having a loving relationship with our parents and siblings. We need to have a set of good friends who understand and support us. As we get married, we also should be considerate of a family of our partner so that we can fully connect with our partner as well as enjoy benefits of the second family.

Engage constantly with family, friends and extended family to stay attached to the roots

Pillar Six: Sky is the Limit

We spend one-third of our day at the workplace. We must be spending it gladly if we want to be happy in life, right? But, it does not happen usually. Sometimes to pay bills, sometimes not to lose pending bonus and promotion, sometimes taking it as a part of every workplace and sometimes to avoid job hunting, we end up ruining our life by going to a workplace that diminishes our happiness.

I was miserable at the office I went to every day. The glittering board of company's name only gave me jitters. The air conditioning of the office that was supposed to regulate the temperature in appropriate ways only suffocated me.

I was adding professional woes to my already troubled life by going to a workplace I no longer love.

Making a choice

From very early on, we are programmed to fall into a profession. Parents view us as a gateway to fulfilling their unachieved ambitions. Teachers take us as a testimony to successfully predict their pupil's fate. We are not allowed to be a part of a profession we would like to spend a part of our lives every day.

We must pause to understand what drives us as a professional. It may sound recital of the script of standard interviews but we actually need to explore and introspect as to where we would like to be after ten years.

It is quite difficult to choose unconventional career paths. We have to be courageous to defy set norms of the society to choose an unusual profession. However, if it makes us happy, it is always worth it to take an offbeat path. Imagine Walt Disney not coming up with cartoons. We would not be having any of beautiful characters of Micky Mouse, Goofy or Snow White. And he has beaten many conventional professionals in terms of both earnings and fame.

Once we have figured out the profession of our choice, our high school and college years can play an important role in laying a foundation of a happy professional life. We can equip ourselves with certifications and skills that are bound to help us in our chosen profession. There are certain skills which are essential across all professions like communication skills, negotiation skills, time management and skill of working in a team. We can also familiarize ourselves with people who are planning to pursue similar professions as us. These strategies will develop us a proficient professional, providing a competitive edge even before we reach the workplace.

Larry page and Sergey Brin are founders of one of the most renowned companies in the world. They created the iconic company Google after they met as classmates while pursuing Ph.D. from Stanford University. Their hard work and diligence at the university led to the development of an idea that went on to revolutionize the way the world searches for information on any topic.

Then, as we reach the golden dais of a workplace after years of schooling and college, we have a tendency to devote ourselves to our bosses. But, it should be our job that should take precedence over any human being. As long as we are honest and diligent in our work, we should not worry about pleasing our bosses or clients.

As observed by Harvard Business Review in its "10 Must Reads" series, workplace requires a plethora of skills that can be developed even before reaching the workplace. And none of these skills relate to appeasing superiors. According to the series, a person's capability to handle conflicts, work well in teams, have innovative thinking and being able to manage emotions are best indicators of his professional caliber.

Switching to betterment

It is only natural to feel comfortable in a setup after a couple of years. We also get used to coming to a particular workplace whether we like it or not after some years. However, we must be willing to keep exploring opportunities to grow in any profession. We must keep our eyes open to grab professional opportunities which will add to our professional achievements.

But, it also happens very often that we continue to be in the same workplace even if we no longer love coming to the same workplace. We continue to be in the same profession even though we do not find ourselves to be a fit for it. It might happen due to societal pressure or our internal weakness that prevent us from seeking perfect profession for us. Similarly, we may continue to do the same job to prevent the hassle of hunting for a job. The idea of drafting a resume, contacting recruiters and going for interviews seem too taxing. We keep on going to the same workplace over and over again, cribbing about the lack of opportunities for us.

According to a news release by Bureau of Labor Statistics (BLS), a unit of United States Department of Labor, an average number of jobs held by baby boomers amounted to 11.7 jobs from age 18 to age 48. It indicates that it was necessary to keep moving to grow professionally even during the era of baby boomers.

Life is too short to be spent doing work we do not enjoy whether it requires a change in profession or a job. It is in our hands to bring about the change that makes us feel contented in whatever we are doing. We should be mindful of time spent at a workplace that does not make us feel energized as it means that we are wasting away our professional aspirations.

Being Dilbert

Even if we are happy with our profession and job, we face such situations at workplace every now and then that throw us off-balance. We all have seen such days at the workplace that does not seem to end, such days that have made us cry more than the worst heartbreak of our life and such days that make us wonder how "Dilbert" is cracking jokes about his workplace.

But, we need to learn to take things in our stride at the workplace. We have to get used to having a full-fledged working life with the need to manage varying expectations in multiple roles. It is altogether a different world with a web of relationships with our colleagues, our boss, and our clients. In addition, we have to walk the tightrope by maintaining the distinction between personal and professional lives.

With different types of pressures weighing us down at the workplace, we must strive to keep our good humor. It is possible only when we take appropriate breaks, spend effective time at the office rather than working long hours, and maintain a healthy lifestyle. It is necessary to keep ourselves light-hearted while managing work so that we can keep on enjoying work during our entire professional life.

Dilbert joke series provides apt humor for every situation of a typical workplace. It talks about the necessity to enjoy pointless meetings, putting up with unnecessary interruptions in work by superiors, superior urging to work extra for no money by utilizing unproductive time in extra work.

I do not dread Monday; I do not wait for Friday (maybe a bit!) when I go to a workplace that fills me with a sense of professional success.

Therefore, it is essential to be happy in whatever profession we choose to be a part of. We can do so by choosing profession/job that makes us feel fulfilled rather than following dictates of society. Also, as in life, we need to keep moving out of our comfort zone to seek opportunities that will shape up our professional life rather than stick to the same workplace. We have to keep our liveliness through a daily dose of humor just like reading cartoon stripes of Dilbert.

Choose a profession wisely and keep updating to achieve professional excellence.

Conclusion

It is very easy to get lost in the daily grind of activities. Our to-do lists take precedence over our long term goals making us wander without a purpose. Our focus on trivial issues makes us lose vision of milestones that has potential to transform our lives for betterment. It is important to keep things in perspective to achieve success in whatever goals we set for ourselves. This book provided a way to keep our path to happiness insight in everyday life.

I hope this book was able to help you to divulge keys to a life full of joy and peace.

And this book enables you to bring about a change in your life as it has brought change in my life. It would also help in bringing improvement in all spheres of your life as it gives a 360-degree view of sources of resentment.

The next step is to actively apply stated strategies in different aspects of our lives so that one day we can look back and only smile!

Made in the USA
Monee, IL
29 August 2023

41835041R00026